C000212608

Heart Failure

Second Edition

Graham Jackson, FRCP
Consultant Cardiologist
Guy's Hospital
London

MARTIN DUNITZ

First published in the United Kingdom in 1991 by
Martin Dunitz Ltd
The Livery House
7−9 Pratt Street
London NW1 0AE

Second edition 1993

ISBN 1 85317 139 5

Typeset by Falcon Graphic Art Ltd
Originated and printed by Toppan Printing
Company (S) Pte Ltd, Singapore

Contents

Introduction   1

Background
Definitions   4
Pathophysiology and terminology   6
Causes of heart failure   10
Clinical presentation   12
Investigations   17

Management
Acute heart failure   20
Chronic heart failure: general advice
  and diuretic therapy   25
Chronic heart failure: vasodilators   32
Inotropic agents   52
Beta-blockers   57
Anticoagulation   58
Anti-arrhythmic drugs   59
Diastolic heart failure   60
Cardiogenic shock   61

Specific Areas
Surgery of heart failure   64
Transplantation   66
Rehabilitation   68
Terminal care   69
Practical points   70

Index   72

For Donald Harrison
and the Class of '78, Cardiology Division, Stanford University,
California

Introduction

The diagnosis and management of heart failure have changed over the last few years. With better detection and treatment of hypertension there is a suggestion that the incidence is falling, but it still represents a major clinical challenge in detection and decision-making.

Echocardiography and Doppler studies now allow us non-invasively to make a quick and accurate diagnosis. Occult valvar disease may be identified and successfully treated, and where the main problem is heart muscle failure angiotensin-converting enzyme (ACE) inhibitors have allowed us to improve quality of life as well as lengthening it.

Heart failure has a poor prognosis with a 50 per cent 5-year and 10 per cent 10-year survival. Over those years it can significantly limit the enjoyment of life. Where the diagnosis is in doubt, or in severe cases, a hospital referral remains in the patient's best interest. An accurate diagnosis can be obtained and the appropriate therapy instituted which can then be translated into out-of-hospital care.

This booklet is intended to be practical and provide a basis for heart failure management in and out of hospital. Our objectives are simple:

- To make the patient feel better

- To enable the patient to do more

- To enable the patient to live longer

- Preferably all of the above

Background

Definitions
Pathophysiology and terminology
Causes of heart failure
Clinical presentation
Investigations

Heart failure

Heart failure occurs when an abnormality of the heart causes cardiac output to fail to meet the body's demands.

The practical manifestations are:

- Acute heart failure

- Chronic heart failure

- Cardiogenic shock (circulatory collapse)

High output failure

Here there is no abnormality of the heart itself as a primary cause, but of course an abnormality may coexist and the high output condition exacerbate or bring out an underlying myocardial problem. High output failure may occur when cardiac output is excessively increased for the following reasons:

- Anaemia

- Thyrotoxicosis

- Paget's disease

- Arteriovenous fistulae (eg, renal dialysis)

- Fever

- Nephritis

- Beriberi

Systolic heart failure

Systolic heart failure occurs when the left ventricle cannot develop enough power to eject blood into the aorta.

The problem is an inability of the muscle to shorten (for example, in primary myocardial disease or secondary to coronary artery disease (CAD)).

Diastolic heart failure

This occurs when the heart muscle is slow to relax so that it cannot accept blood and fill at low diastolic pressures.

The problem is increased chamber stiffness (for example, in hypertensive heart disease, CAD, hypertrophic cardiomyopathy).

Left heart failure

A clinical diagnosis relating to left-sided, usually left ventricular (LV), failure and manifested clinically as the symptoms of pulmonary congestion (dyspnoea, orthopnoea and paroxysmal nocturnal dyspnoea (PND)).

Right heart failure

A clinical diagnosis implying right-sided (right ventricular) failure, manifested clinically as hepatic congestion, raised venous pressure, peripheral oedema and ascites. In most cases the marked fluid retention observed reflects poor renal perfusion due to LV failure rather than failure of the right ventricle itself. This is why right and left heart failure most often coexist.

Pathophysiology and terminology

The principal determinants of cardiac function are:

- Preload
- Afterload
- Contractility
- Heart rate and rhythm

Cardiac output

This is the stroke volume (volume of blood ejected with each heart beat) multiplied by the heart rate:

$$CO = SV \times HR.$$

As output falls the rate will rise usually due to sympathetic nervous system activation. Sinus tachycardia which is unexplained may be an early sign of heart failure.

Neurohumoral changes

With developing failure the effective blood volume declines, and activation of the sympathetic nervous system, renin–angiotensin system and arginine vasopressin (AVP) attempts to reverse this (see below).

Other changes may antagonize these vasoconstrictors. Plasma atrial natriuretic factor (ANF) which can cause vasodilatation and diuresis may be elevated, but the clinical effect is variable and limited. Prostaglandins PGE_2 and PGI_2 are activated and may antagonize the vasoconstriction as well as act with angiotensin II to maintain glomerular filtration by dilating afferent glomerular arterioles, in contrast to the efferent arteriole constriction caused by angiotensin II. Agents which inhibit prostaglandins must be used cautiously (for example, non-steroidal anti-inflammatory agents).

Preload

This is the volume of blood present in the left ventricle at the end of diastole, that is, immediately before ejection. This can also be expressed in terms of the degree of stretch experienced by the LV muscle as a result of the volume of blood at the end of diastole. With higher volumes there should be greater stretch-

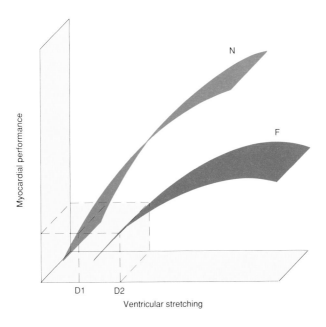

Figure 1

Ventricular function curves. The normal curve (N) contrasts with the failing heart (F). The function curve is depressed by a fall in contractility (N to F). In terminal failure the curve is down-sloping. In the normal heart a unit increase in preload (D1) leads to a unit increase in output, but the failing heart has a greater degree of stretch and a less significant rise in output (D2).

ing and a greater volume of blood ejected (Figure 1). If ventricular function is depressed the response is impaired and, whereas for each unit increase in preload there should be a similar unit increase in output, this response fails. With the failure to clear volume, pressures increase (the left ventricular end-diastolic pressure, LVEDP), these are transmitted to the lungs and back-pressure failure ensues (pulmonary congestion, dyspnoea).

The mechanisms responsible for increased preload include salt and water retention from a reduction in cardiac output, affecting the renin−angiotensin system, and increased sympathetic tone. The former leads to angiotensin activation, aldosterone production, salt and water reabsorption by the kidney and vasoconstriction: the latter to reduced venous capacitance, venoconstriction, increased venous return and also increased peripheral resistance (Figure 2). Thus the short-term gain of an attempt to increase myocardial stretching also increases capillary pressure (congestion), which is usually the prominent feature of heart failure.

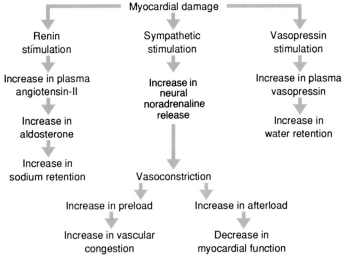

Figure 2
Neurohormonal activation after myocardial damage: the vicious circle of heart failure.

Afterload

This is an expression of the force the heart muscle must generate to overcome the resistance to blood flow in the aorta (aortic impedance) and the peripheral arteries (peripheral resistance) — in other words, the total peripheral resistance. Afterload is increased secondary to increased preload as a consequence of ventricular dilatation, activation of the renin–angiotensin system and sympathetic stimulation. Increased afterload increases the work required to pump blood around the body and is therefore liable to impair further the performance of the failing ventricle.

Contractility

This refers to the force of ventricular contraction independent of loading; that is, it is intrinsic to the contractile proteins actin and myosin which are found in the thick and thin filaments of the myocardial sarcomere. Calcium is essential for cardiac contraction. An increase in activation of the sympathetic nervous system increases heart rate and helps maintain the contractile state, but at the expense of increasing preload, afterload and oxygen demand. The more severe the failure, the greater the level of circulatory catecholamines — a response akin to 'flogging a dead horse'.

In most cases, heart failure is due to systolic failure. Preload and afterload increase, and failure is termed 'compensated' when output is maintained.

Decompensated heart failure occurs when the body's intrinsic ability fails. As afterload and preload further increase, the compensatory mechanism becomes counterproductive, adding further to the load of the failing heart. A vicious circle develops — failure begets failure — and it is our job to interrupt this chain of events.

Causes of heart failure

Direct myocardial damage

- CAD
- Cardiomyopathies
- Myocarditis
- Alcohol

Volume overload

- Aortic regurgitation
- Mitral regurgitation
- Post-infarction ventricular septal defect (VSD)
- Atrial septal defect

Pressure overload

- Aortic stenosis
- Hypertension
- Coarctation of aorta

Impaired ventricular filling

- Mitral stenosis

- Constrictive pericarditis

- Hypertrophic cardiomyopathy

- Restrictive cardiomyopathy

- Atrial myxoma

Precipitating causes

- Arrhythmias, particularly atrial fibrillation (AF) with a rapid ventricular rate

- Infection, especially pneumonia in the elderly

- Thyrotoxicosis

- Anaemia, again more frequently in the elderly

- Bacterial endocarditis

- Beta-blockade

- Calcium antagonists

- Anti-arrhythmic drugs (eg, flecainide, disopyramide)

- Non-steroidal anti-inflammatory agents

- Steroids

- Doxorubicin

- Lithium

Clinical presentation

Acute heart failure

A sudden event leads to abrupt deterioration of LV function. The commonest causes are:

- CAD (usually a myocardial infarct)

- Arrhythmias (frequently AF)

Acute heart failure may occur on the background of chronic heart failure. The findings are:

- Severe breathlessness

- Pulmonary oedema

- Cyanosis

- Peripheral vasoconstriction

Chronic heart failure

A chronic condition reflected in symptoms and signs by the effects of a low cardiac output with retention of sodium and water. The degree of limitation has been graded by the New York Heart Association (Table 1) on practical but somewhat subjective assessments of exercise ability.

Breathlessness

This is the most common complaint, usually reflecting a preload problem. Breathlessness may be worse at night when lying flat (orthopnoea) and can wake the patient when PND occurs. This reflects nocturnal absorption of fluid at a time of decreased awareness (sleep) and classically leads to gasping respiration,

Table 1
NYHA classification

Class I	Patients with cardiac disease but with no limitation during ordinary physical activity
Class II	Slight limitations caused by cardiac disease. Activity such as walking causes dyspnoea
Class III	Marked limitation. Symptoms are provoked easily, for example, by walking on flat ground.
Class IV	Breathlessness at rest

coughing and wheezing sometimes with frothy sputum. The patient gains relief from sitting up or standing and may even sleep in a chair for fear of it occurring.

Whilst it is usual to associate breathlessness with heart failure or respiratory disease, the patient may feel the ache in the chest or tightening constriction of angina as a form of breathlessness. It is important to ask 'what do you mean by breathlessness?' — a surprising number may say 'tightness', have no systolic dysfunction and be suffering from angina rather than heart failure, with important therapeutic implications.

Fatigue and lethargy

These can be considered as afterload problems or forward failure. Lack of output may reduce cerebral blood flow, causing confusion or slowness of thought, and skeletal muscle flow, inducing fatigue, heavy legs and lethargy. The patient may express this in a variety of ways — 'no life in me', 'everything's an effort', or 'all I want to do is sleep'.

Oedema

Swollen ankles are what patients most often complain of and are worse at the end of the day. Older people often do not mention the oedema until it is severe, even above the knees. Increased right heart pressures which are the cause may also distend the liver (right hypochondrial pain) and lead to bowel oedema and/or ascites (bloated abdomen, loss of appetite).

Table 2
Symptoms and signs of heart failure

Symptoms	Shortness of breath	Fatigue
	Swollen ankles	Wheezing
	Tired out	Cough at night
	Need to sit out of bed	Painful abdomen
	Need to open windows for air	Anorexia
	Swollen abdomen	

Signs	Breathless easily (undressing)	Jugular venous pressure raised
	Wheeze audible	Ankle oedema
	Tachycardia	Tender large liver
	Third or fourth sound (or both)	Ascites
		Cardiomegaly
	Basal crackles	Murmurs

Examination

The principal signs of cardiac failure are:

- Tachycardia

- Cardiomegaly

- Third or fourth heart sounds or both

- A raised jugular venous pressure (JVP)

- Basal crackles

- Peripheral oedema

Not all need be present at any one time.

Invariably there is a sinus tachycardia with or without extrasystoles, and in more chronic cases AF is frequent. An acute deterioration in a previously stable patient may be due to the sudden onset of AF with a rapid ventricular response and this must always be excluded. Blood pressure may be high or low, depending on the aetiology (for example, hypertension) and state of LV function.

Third and fourth heart sounds are best heard at the apex with the stethoscope bell lightly applied and the patient on his left side. When both are present the heart appears to gallop. The commonest lung signs are basal crackles, but wheezes and a pleural effusion may also be present. The effusion can be unilateral as well as bilateral (no air entry, dull to percussion).

It is vitally important when examining the heart failure patient to answer the following questions:

Is this really heart failure?

Could it be angina? Could it be a primary respiratory problem? Is the patient anxious, worried and hyperventilating, and are you sure there is nothing to suggest diabetes?

If it is failure — is there a reason?

The prognosis of heart muscle failure is poor, so we need to exclude a mechanical cause. Is there any evidence of valvar pathology? When output is low, murmurs will be soft so they must not be dismissed as 'functional' without echocardiography. In ischaemic patients listen for the harsh mitral regurgitant murmur of papillary muscle dysfunction (apex to back) and always think of aortic valve disease. Remember too that alcohol on its own can cause heart failure, and a detailed history is needed.

Is there a non-cardiac cause?

Look for evidence of anaemia and severe infection, especially in older patients. Is there evidence of thyrotoxicosis? Check the drug therapy, in particular beta-blockers, calcium antagonists, non-steroidal anti-inflammatory agents, salt-containing antacids

and carbenoxalone. An older patient who is breathless may
have other problems, and neoplasia with hepatic secondaries
should always be considered.

Cardiogenic shock

This is characterized by:

- Pallor

- Systolic blood pressure (SBP) < 90 mm Hg

- Cold clammy extremities

- Oliguria (< 20 ml/hr)

- Cerebral hypoperfusion (confusion)

The commonest cause is acute myocardial infarction but the
following must also be considered:

- Pulmonary embolus (any evidence of deep venous thrombosis (DVT)?)

- Tamponade (recent cardiac operation or procedure,
  trauma, infarction, viral illness?)

- Septicaemia (acute endocarditis)

- Haemorrhage (peptic ulcer, ruptured aneurysm)

- Acute right ventricular infarction (infarct presentation,
  usually inferior and/or posterior changes, JVP raised but
  lungs clear)

- Diabetic ketoacidosis

- Drug overdose

Chest radiograph

This should be routine and can be used to monitor therapy, although changes in the radiograph often lag behind clinical improvement. If the transverse diameter of the heart is greater than 15.5 cm in the man and 14.5 cm in the woman there is cardiomegaly. When the pulmonary venous pressure rises (normal ‹ 15 mm Hg), first the upper zone veins become dilated (› 3 mm diameter) — 'upper zone blood vessel dilatation'. As the pulmonary pressure increases (usually above 20 mm Hg) Kerley lines appear, and finally (at greater than 25 mm Hg) pulmonary oedema and pleural effusions.

The chest radiograph can also identify valvar calcification, suggest a LV aneurysm or rarely pick up pericardial calcification.

ECG

There are no specific ECG features of heart failure but the ECG establishes the rhythm, the presence or absence of LV hypertrophy and documents evidence of infarction and sometimes ischaemia. A normal ECG does not equate invariably with a normal heart and can be dangerously reassuring. A 24-hour ECG is essential if arrhythmias are suspected.

Echocardiography

It is my routine policy to perform an echocardiogram on all patients undergoing therapy for heart failure. While it may establish the diagnosis of a myopathic ventricle it also excludes significant suspected or unsuspected valvar pathology which can be quantified with Doppler. Echocardiography may identify a significant and operable LV aneurysm as well as intracavity thrombus. The presence of echocardiographic global LV dysfunction will preclude the need for diagnostic angiography, and Doppler assessment of valvar incompetence will avoid unnecessary angiography to assess the functional significance of a murmur in the presence of severe LV dysfunction. Echocardiography will identify pericardial effusions and any localized wall-movement abnormalities reflecting right or left ventricular infarction.

In a minority of patients echocardiography identifies a primary abnormality of diastolic rather than systolic function.

Angiography

This is reserved for cases of diagnostic doubt or uncertainty as to whether there is a mechanical problem that can be corrected. This is now only necessary in a small number of cases, due to the developments in echocardiography and colour-flow Doppler. Angiography remains essential for the evaluation of the coronary arteries.

Pathology

- Full blood count

- Urea and electrolytes (U & E), creatinine and blood glucose

- Liver function tests

- Thyroid function tests if diagnostic doubts

- Cardiac enzymes if infarct queried

- Blood cultures if endocarditis suspected

Management

Acute heart failure
Chronic heart failure:
general advice and diuretic therapy
Chronic heart failure: vasodilators
Inotropic agents
Beta-blockers
Anticoagulation
Anti-arrhythmic drugs
Diastolic heart failure
Cardiogenic shock

Acute heart failure

This is a medical emergency and implies LV dysfunction leading to pulmonary oedema. Rarely these days the presentation is secondary to mitral stenosis or, extremely rarely, a left atrial myxoma. Mitral stenosis should always be considered in younger women, particularly from Middle and Far Eastern countries. Mitral stenotic murmurs and increasing dyspnoea in the presence of sinus rhythm is a left atrial myxoma until proved otherwise by urgent echocardiography.

Management

- Patients are usually more comfortable sitting up.

- Order investigations (Table 3).

- Oxygen 8 l/min safety-mask or 4 l/min MC mask. 25 per cent if chronic obstructive airways disease (COAD).

- Diamorphine 2.5–5 mg iv or morphine 5–10 mg iv over 3–5 minutes. Use antiemetic (eg, cyclizine 50 mg iv, prochlorperazine 12.5 mg im). Avoid opiates (out of hospital) if COAD: cautious use in hospital (have naloxone 0.4 mg iv available).

- Frusemide 40–80 mg iv or bumetanide 1–2 mg iv. Immediate benefit from vasodilatation, then diuresis in 5–30 minutes. Beware elderly male prostates — risk of urinary retention. If renal failure, try frusemide effusion 250 mg iv over 1 hour, request renal opinion (dialysis may be necessary). If desperate, venesect 500 cc or rotate cuffs on legs to isolate blood volume for 30 minutes each.

Table 3
Urgent investigations

ECG	Rhythm? Infarct?
Chest radiograph	Confirms oedema + effusion; excludes pneumonia, pneumothorax
Urea and electrolytes	Renal status + potassium and glucose
Blood count	Anaemia?
Echocardiogram	Urgent if mechanical cause suspected or no obvious reason

Nitrates

Nitrates used out of hospital sublingually and in hospital intravenously or orally act by reducing preload.

- Glyceryl trinitrate (GTN) 0.5 mg sublingual × 1 or 2

- GTN spray sublingual × 2

- Isosorbide mononitrate 20 mg bid oral

- Isosorbide dinitrate (ISDN) iv 2−10 mg/hr; titrate but keep SBP ›90 mm Hg

- or GTN iv 10-200 μg/min

Aminophylline

- Especially if bronchospasm

- 250 mg iv over 10 min

- Not if on oral theophyllines (toxicity more likely − arrhythmias)

Digoxin

- Only if AF with rapid ventricular rate

- Check potassium

- In hospital digoxin 1 mg iv over 1 hour, then oral regime (usually 0.25 mg daily)

Follow-up

Repeat frusemide 40−80 mg iv if residual oedema, then establish oral regime.

If low output:
1 commence dopamine 5 μg/kg per minute (renal dose) plus dobutamine 5−25 μg/kg per minute. Titrate cautiously to avoid excessive tachycardia or arrhythmias. Monitor effect on SBP response (aim for 110−120 mm Hg) and diuresis (>30 ml/hr).

2 Insert Swan–Ganz catheter to monitor pulmonary artery (PA) pressures and arterial line. Ideally do this before (1), but in the real world delay may occur whilst equipment is assembled.

3 Manage as cardiogenic shock (page 61−2).

Identify cause:
1 History — Has there been recent chest pain?
       — Does the patient take cardiac drugs or have a preceding cardiac condition?

2 ECG — Any evidence of recent infarction?
    — Check the rhythm

3 Echocardiogram — What is the LV status?
            — Is there any evidence of a significant valvar lesion?

4 Pathology — anaemia?
       — renal dysfunction?
       — diabetic?

Is there a mechanical solution (eg, ruptured mitral cusp, post-infarct VSD, aortic valve disease)? If so, refer to surgeons for an immediate opinion.

Is AF present (or do you strongly suspect it occurred — is there a history of rapid palpitations?)? If so:

1 Digoxin, iv or oral depending on status. If in AF with rapid ventricular rate — iv, then oral. If SR and history or evidence of intermittent AF − oral. Make sure K^+ normal.

2 Anticoagulate initially with heparin 30 000 units/day, then warfarin. Target INR (international normalized ratio) 2.0−3.0.

3 Consider immediate DC shock if AF recent and hypotension continues. Check LV first, administer heparin 10 000 units iv. Digoxin not an increased risk, but begin with 100 Joules.

4 Exclude thyrotoxicosis, especially if LV satisfactory on echo.

5 Remember alcohol history.

6 If AF control poor (rate ›100) and digitalization completed. In the presence of systolic failure and LV dysfunction, commence oral amiodarone 400 mg tds 2 days, 200 mg tds 5 days, then 200 mg daily. Remember amiodarone potentiates digoxin levels. Alternatively, infuse amiodarone 300 mg (5 mg/kg) in 5 per cent dextrose over 30 minutes via a central vein if possible (thrombophlebitis risk). Begin oral regime at 200 mg tds but also continue to give up to 1200 mg iv (ie, 15 mg/kg) over 24 hours.

7 If AF control poor and echo shows diastolic dysfunction with good systolic function, begin beta-blockade once failure controlled or minimal residual problem. Consider

xamoterol 200 mg, atenolol 25 mg or propranolol 10 mg as starting test doses. Alternatively, calcium antagonists diltiazem 30−60 mg tds and verapamil 40−80 mg tds.

Is LV function substantially impaired? If so, manage as chronic failure.

Table 4
Digitalization

Urgent	1 mg iv over 1 hour, then 0.25 mg orally daily
Routine	0.5 mg tds 1 day orally, then 0.25 mg daily
Rapid	0.5 mg iv, then oral 0.25 mg twice day, then 0.25 mg daily
Maintenance	Normal: 0.25 mg daily — judge clinically Creatinine clearance 10−25 ml/min: 0.125 mg daily, and monitor levels Age >70 years: 0.125 mg−0.25 mg daily — judge on effect, check levels if necessary Age >70 years and renal dysfunction: 0.0625−0.125 mg daily. Monitor levels
Therapeutic range	0.8−2.0 ng/ml (1.0−2.6 nmol/l) Blood taken 6 hours post dose Check K^+ at same time (page 53).

Table 5
Acute heart failure therapy

Out of hospital	Sit up Oxygen if available (25 per cent COAD) Frusemide 80 mg iv Aminophylline 250 mg iv if bronchospasm severe: slow injection over 10 minutes Sublingual nitrates 0.5 mg × 2 or spray Morphine/antiemetic.
In hospital	Try to identify causes as quickly as possible If circulatory collapse, manage as for shock (page 47) If stabilizing, continue diuretics and vasodilators Digoxin for AF Consider anticoagulants

Chronic heart failure: general advice and diuretic therapy

General measures

Initially:

- Bed or chair rest if severe failure
- Gentle leg exercises to help prevent DVT
- Avoid constipation (diuretics dehydrate the bowel; straining drops cardiac output)
- Stop smoking
- Abstain from alcohol
- Reduce salt.

When stabilized:

- Alcohol 1—2 units a day unless the primary cause of the failure
- Maintain optimum weight
- Social, environmental counselling (housing etc)
- Advice on exercise, avoiding isometrics (see page 68)
- Emphasize importance of compliance

Assuming we have removed any underlying cause, we are left with treating heart failure due to left ventricular systolic dysfunction. I shall deal with diastolic dysfunction separately.

Drug therapy

The principle

Should we stimulate the heart (digoxin) or unload it (diuretics, vasodilators) or both? Our current approach in the presence of sinus rhythm is to unload the heart first of all, but when there is cardiomegaly and a gallop rhythm, and these options have been employed, digoxin is now of proven additional value.

We want to reduce congestion (breathlessness) but not to dehydrate; we want to facilitate output by reducing afterload but not to reduce the blood pressure too far, and then to increase contractility if necessary (see Figure 3).

In addition, we want to lengthen life by using drugs that not only perform some of these duties but also have few adverse effects, which in practice means using ACE inhibitors as soon as possible.

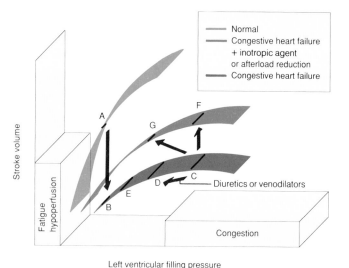

Figure 3
The principle of heart failure therapy.

As shown before (see Figure 1), patients with myocardial damage have a depressed LV function curve. When the stroke volume falls (A → B) preload is increased because of fluid retention and venoconstriction (B → C). Increased levels of circulating catecholamines may increase contractility (C → F). Diuretics and venodilators reduce filling pressure (preload) without any significant effect on output (stroke volume). If the curve is flat, movement will be from C to D, but too great a reduction will take the preload from D to E. At this point the curve is still rising, so to dry out the patient too much will actually cause output to fall. Agents that reduce afterload or improve contractility result in movement from C to F, whereas to add preload reduction to afterload reduction obtains the best of both mechanisms — C to G (that is, less congestion, more output).

Diuretics

- Drugs of choice in the presence of fluid retention

- Frequent clinical assessment because of variable individual needs until stable

- U & E
    1. Urea rising may reflect over-diuresis
    2. Keep K^+ >3.5 mmol/l
    3. If frusemide >160 mg/day, monitor calcium and magnesium

- Diuretics reduce preload and breathlessness. They have no major impact on exercise ability nor do they lengthen life.

Thiazides

- More effective in mild failure

- Act on distal tubule

- Gentle action, begin at 1 hour, peak at 4 and last 10−12 hours

- Socially convenient

- Fewer prostatic problems

- More tendency to hypokalaemia than loop agents.

Loop diuretics

- Act on the ascending limb of loop of Henle

- Weak effect on convoluted tubule also

- Rapid action, iv in 5 minutes, orally 1 hour, peak 2 hours, duration 4−6 hours

- Frusemide 40 mg equal to bumetanide 1 mg

- Can be used with thiazides for additive effect

- Cause hypokalaemia.

Potassium-sparing agents

- *Spironolactone* inhibits aldosterone in the distal tubule

- Useful with hepatic congestion (secondary aldosteronism especially if JVP >12 cm)

- Onset 48−72 hours (hypokalaemia may occur earlier therefore). Effect can increase over weeks, leading to overdiuresis

- Painful gynaecomastia in men can be a problem

- *Amiloride* and *triamterene* act independently of aldosterone, and gynaecomastia is not a significant problem

- Beware of hyperkalaemia if renal impairment with any potassium-sparing agent

- Beware of hyperkalaemia if co-prescribing with ACE inhibitors

- Beware of hyponatraemia, especially in the elderly.

Choice of diuretic

Mild failure:

- Thiazide
    1 Bendrofluazide 5−10 mg daily if adequate diet. Monitor U & E. Consider captopril also.
    2 Potassium-sparing agent (hydrochlorothiazide 25 mg, plus triamterene 50 mg) one or two daily. Caution in the elderly.

- Loop diuretic: frusemide 20−40 mg or bumetanide 0.5−1 mg daily, consider captopril at the same time. Or combination (potassium-sparing) with amiloride once daily. Bumetanide may be less diabetogenic than frusemide. Monitor U & E.
  NB Digoxin if in AF
  NB Bendrofluazide 10 mg, equivalent to frusemide 20 mg

Moderate heart failure:

- Loop diuretic as above. Frusemide 40–80 mg or bumetanide 1–2 mg once or twice daily, plus ACE inhibitor or frusemide 40 mg plus amiloride 5 mg daily (no more than two a day). Monitor U & E.

Severe heart failure:

- If gross oedema use iv loop agents to guarantee bioavailability (eg, frusemide 80 mg iv or more)

- Frusemide oral 40–80 mg or bumetanide 1–2 mg once or twice daily, thereafter increasing as necessary

- But do not increase dose without also considering ACE inhibitors

- Potassium-sparing agents in addition or combination, eg frusemide 40 mg plus amiloride 5 mg up to twice daily or frusemide plus spironolactone (frusemide 80 mg + spironolactone 50 mg). Beware hyperkalaemia if ACE inhibitors in use

- Regular checks on U & E until patient stable

- Monitor effect on daily weight 1 kg = 1 litre; aim to lose 0.5 kg/day.

Resistant oedema:

- Institute iv therapy

- Change iv loop (eg, switch from frusemide to bumetanide)

- Change oral loop (eg, frusemide 80 mg to bumetanide 2 mg once or twice daily and titrate)

- Add metolazone 5–10 mg daily (response can be dramatic)

- Add bendrofluazide 5–10 mg daily as alternative to metolazone

- Avoid overdiuresis. Keep JVP 1 cm above sternal notch with patient at 90 degrees. JVP should be visible with the patient lying flat. Some residual ankle oedema is often necessary to maintain right ventricular filling pressure

Diuretic side-effects:

- Hypokalaemia (potentiates digoxin side-effects)

- Hyperkalaemia if renal impairment and potassium-sparing agent used or potassium-sparing agent and ACE inhibitor

- Hyponatraemia in a waterlogged patient
    1 Restrict fluid to 1000 ml/day
    2 Use vasodilators and inotropes temporarily
    3 In the elderly this may occur unpredictably with amiloride (weakness, nausea, confusion) and they may also be dry (see below)

- Hyponatraemia in a dehydrated patient
    1 Stop all agents (usually loop diuretics)
    2 Check K^+, may be high
    3 Slowly rehydrate with normal saline up to 1500 ml/day
    4 Reintroduce diuretics cautiously as fluid volume increases and consider ACE inhibitors early
    5 Regular U & Es essential

- Hyperuricaemia. Care is needed using indomethacin for acute gout as failure may be worsened. Colchicine an alternative (1 mg initially, then 500 μg 3-hourly until pain relief or vomiting and diarrhoea. Maximum dose 10 mg. Repeat course if needed in 3 days). Allopurinol may be needed long term (100−300 mg daily)

- Glucose intolerance
    1 May resolve when hypokalaemia corrected
    2 The elderly are vulnerable
    3 Diabetics may slip out of control
    4 Needs regular monitoring

Chronic heart failure: vasodilators

Vasodilators can be used to reduce preload by dilating venous capacitance vessels or afterload by dilating arterioles. Patients whose symptoms reflect increased preload (venous congestion) should respond better to a venodilator, while patients with depressed LV function and symptoms of low output should respond better to an arteriolar dilator. However, as the two conditions must often go together a drug with both properties — a balanced vasodilator, or a mixture of venous and arterial dilators — should be the most effective. Table 6 lists the important oral and intravenous vasodilators.

In the past vasodilators tended to be reserved for the more severe cases of heart failure but their earlier use is likely to lead to lower diuretic dosage and an improved quality of life. In this way it may be possible to down titrate diuretic dosage.

Table 6
Vasodilators used in the treatment of heart failure

Agent	Site of action Arterial	Venous	Mode of administration	Duration of action
Nitroglycerin	*	**	Sublingual, intravenous, topical	Minutes to hours
ISDN	*	**	Sublingual, oral, intravenous	Minutes to hours
Isosorbide mononitrate	*	**	Oral	Hours
Hydralazine	**	*	Oral	Hours
ACE inhibitors	**	*	Oral	Hours
Flosequinan	**	**	Oral	Hours

* = minor action
** = major action

A series of major and important studies have now been published which show clear-cut mortality and morbidity benefits from vasodilators across the spectrum of heart failure from asymptomatic LV dysfunction to class IV failure. All trials are concerned with systolic pump failure.

Veterans Administration Vasodilator Heart (V-He FT I) Trial

Background:

- Moderate–severe heart failure (NYHA II–IV)

- Standard therapy of digoxin and diuretic

- Placebo, prazosin or hydralazine plus ISDN added

Results:

- 34 per cent decrease in mortality on hydralazine and ISDN compared to placebo (34.3–25.6 per cent) at two years (Figure 4)

- Prazosin not different from placebo

- LV ejection fraction improved on hydralazine and ISDN

- Side-effects common with hydralazine and ISDN – only 55 per cent able to take full doses at 6 months (hydralazine 50 mg tds, ISDN 60 mg tds)

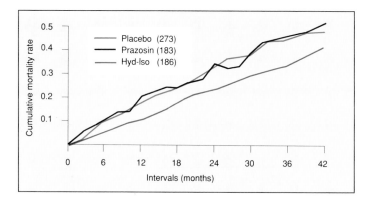

Figure 4
Mortality-risk reduction in patients
treated with ISDN and hydralazine
for mild–moderate failure.

(Reproduced with permission from
N Engl J Med *(1986)* **314**: *1550.)*

Co-operative North Scandinavian Enalapril Survival Study (CONSENSUS)

Background:

- Severe heart failure (NYHA IV)

- Enalapril (up to 40 mg daily) vs placebo added to digoxin and diuretics

Results:

- 27 per cent reduction in mortality on enalapril at 1 year (52–36 per cent) (Figure 5)

- Improved symptoms and signs of failure

- Side-effects (withdrawals) similar to placebo (that is, well tolerated)

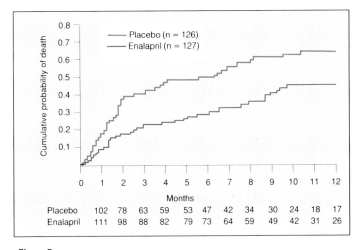

	0	1	2	3	4	5	6	7	8	9	10	11	12
Placebo		102	78	63	59	53	47	42	34	30	24	18	17
Enalapril		111	98	88	82	79	73	64	59	49	42	31	26

Figure 5
Mortality in the Co-operative North Scandinavian
Enalapril Survival Study (CONSENSUS).
(Reproduced with permission from N Engl J Med (1987) **316:**
1431.)

V-HeFT II

Background:

- Compared enalapril up to 20 mg with hydralazine up to
  300 mg and ISDN up to 160 mg daily added to conventional
  therapy

- Mild–moderate failure (NHYA II–III)

Results:

- Mortality at 2 years on enalapril 18 per cent and hydralazine
  plus ISDN 25 per cent ($P = 0.016$) (Figure 6)

- Less sudden death on enalapril but similar pump failure.
  Hydralazine/ISDN produced greater improvement in exercise
  ability and LV ejection fraction

- Suggests a role for combination therapy

- Enalapril better tolerated than hydralazine plus ISDN with improved functional status

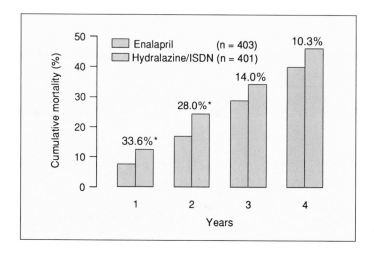

Figure 6
Effects of vasodilators on mortality in the V-HeFT II trial. Statistically significant mortality differences between treatment groups are asterisked. (Reproduced with permission from N Engl J Med (1991) 325:309.)

Studies of Left Ventricular Dysfunction (SOLVD)

Background:

- Enalapril up to 20 mg daily vs placebo in chronic LV dysfunction (42 months)

- Two groups, one with mild−moderate heart failure (NYHA II and III) (treatment trial) and the other with asymptomatic LV dysfunction (prevention trial)

- Prevention trial included 80 per cent with previous myocardial infarction, but not within 30 days (average 1 year) − a different group from the SAVE trial

Results of treatment trial:

- 16 per cent reduction in risk of death on enalapril (39.7 − 35.2 per cent, $P = 0.0036$) (Figure 7) at 2 years

- Reduced progression of failure

- Fewer hospital admissions (risk reduction of 26 per cent)

- Better quality of life

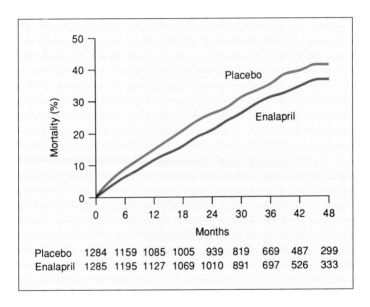

Figure 7

*Mortality curves in the placebo and enalapril groups in SOLVD. The numbers of patients alive in each group at the end of each period are shown at the bottom of the figure. (Reproduced with permission from N Eng J Med (1991) **325**: 296.)*

Results of prevention trial:

- Mortality risk reduced by 8 per cent (NS)

- When heart failure development is added to mortality risk the reduction on enalapril was 29 per cent, $P < 0.001$ (Figure 8)

- Fewer hospital admissions for heart failure on enalapril (risk reduction 20 per cent, $P < 0.001$)

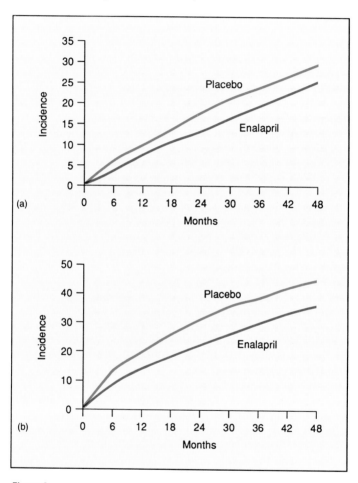

Figure 8
(a) Death or hospitalization for congestive heart failure and (b) death or development of heart failure in the SOLVD prevention trial. (Reproduced with permission from N Engl J Med (1992) 327: 688.)

Survival and Ventricular Enlargement (SAVE) Trial

Background:

- Reduced LV function *without* symptoms 3–16 days post infarction (asymptomatic LV dysfunction)

- No symptoms of ischaemia

- Captopril up to 50 mg tds vs placebo (42 months)

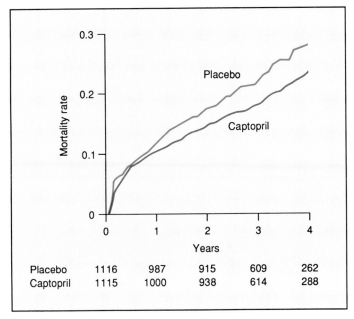

Figure 9
Cumulative mortality from all causes in the study groups. The number of patients at risk at the beginning of each year is shown at the bottom. (Reproduced with permission from N Engl J Med (1992) 327: 672.)

Results:

- All-cause mortality reduced by 19 per cent, $P = 0.019$ (Figure 9)

- Reduced fatal and non-fatal cardiovascular events (21 per cent, $P = 0.014$ death; 37 per cent, $P < 0.001$ for development of severe heart failure; and 25 per cent for recurrent myocardial infarction, $P = 0.015$) (Figure 10)

- Additive to all other therapies (eg, thrombolysis, aspirin, beta-blockade etc)

- Adverse effects similar on captopril and placebo (ie, captopril well tolerated)

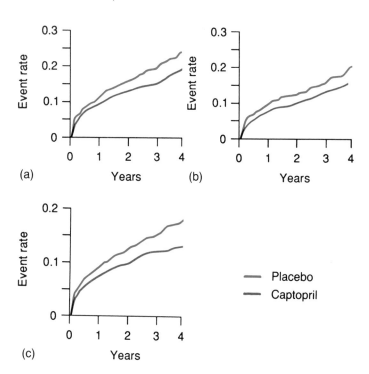

Figure 10

Life-tables for cumulative fatal and non-fatal cardiovascular events: (a) death from cardiovascular events; (b) congestive heart failure requiring ACE inhibitors; (c) recurrent myocardial infarction. (Reproduced with permission from N Engl J Med (1992) 327: 673.)

Munich Mild Heart Failure Trial

Background:

- Mild heart failure (NYHA II)

- Captopril 25 mg bid vs placebo added to conventional therapy

- Followed for 2.7 years

Results:

- Captopril reduced progression to severe heart failure from 26.4 per cent on placebo to 10.8 per cent ($P = 0.01$)

- Not a mortality study but when death and progression of failure are combined the reduction was from 32.4 per cent on placebo to 14.0 per cent on captopril (Figure 11)

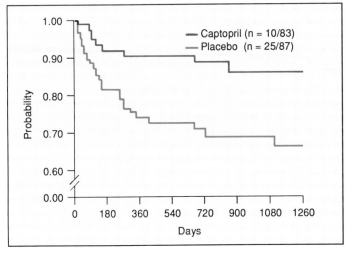

Figure 11
*Prognostic implications of ACE inhibitors in patients with mild heart failure. The probability (Kaplan-Meier estimate) of being free of pump failure (NYHA IV) or death in pump failure is indicated on the vertical axis. (Reproduced with permission from Z Kardiol (1990) **79** (Suppl 1): 149A.)*

HY-C Trial

Background:

- Captopril vs hydralazine plus ISDN added to conventional therapy

- Titrated to achieve same haemodynamic effects as judged by wedge pressure at Swan−Ganz catheterization

Results:

- Actuarial 1-year survival: 81 per cent on captopril and 51 per cent on hydralazine ($P = 0.05$) (Figure 12)

- Reduced sudden death with captopril ($P = 0.01$)

- Only trial to titrate to objective degree of vasodilatation

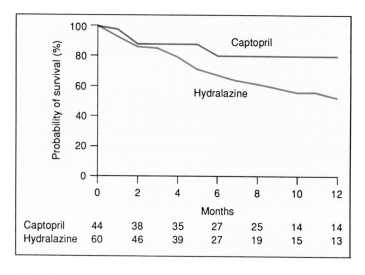

Figure 12
Kaplan-Meier survival curves for the 104 patients discharged on the oral vasodilator regime of captopril or hydralazine plus ISDN.

*(Reproduced with permission from JACC (1992) **19**: 846.)*

Summary

These trials have established the need for and usefulness of vasodilators in the management of heart failure, and the advantages of ACE inhibitors in terms of improving quality and quantity of life are clear-cut.

We can conclude:

- ACE inhibitors should be considered at *all* stages of symptomatic heart failure. They improve quantity and quality of life.

- ACE inhibitors are also beneficial in the presence of asymptomatic LV dysfunction, with or without recent infarction.

- Higher doses of ACE inhibitors should be used than is current practice; eg, captopril 25 mg bd or tds and 50 mg bid or tds.

- The efficacy of ACE inhibitors may be improved by the co-prescription of oral nitrates which are likely to maximize the haemodynamic benefits.

- When ACE inhibitors are contraindicated or induce adverse effects the hydralazine/ISDN combination is a valuable alternative.

- Adverse effects are not a major limitation to use (ie, they are well tolerated).

Angiotensin-converting enzyme inhibitors

ACE inhibitors have properties additional to vasodilatation alone but are classed here for simplicity (see Table 7).

These drugs have many desirable properties for the management of heart failure. They act by interfering with the renin−angiotensin system (Figure 13). They reduce aldosterone production (a diuretic effect) and act as vasodilators. Their proven beneficial effects are:

- Dyspnoea is reduced

- Exercise is increased

- Hospital care is reduced

- Life expectancy is extended in all grades of heart failure

Approximately 70 per cent of patients with chronic heart failure respond to ACE inhibitors symptomatically. They must not be introduced to the dehydrated patient or to severe heart failure patients out of hospital. They can be carefully initiated out of hospital under supervision in mild to moderate cases. It is vitally important that practical guidelines are followed in order to avoid adverse effects. These are drugs which must be given to the right patients correctly at the right time.

- The diagnosis must be established.

- There must be no evidence of significant valvar stenosis.

- Check U & E normal or only mildly impaired (urea < 12.0 mmol/l).

- Check the patient is not dry: can you see JVP in the patient lying flat?

- Check the SBP is >100 mm Hg.

- Consider at frusemide 40 mg or equivalent and above.

- Warn of the first dose's hypotensive effect. Take it sitting, relaxing or just before bed.

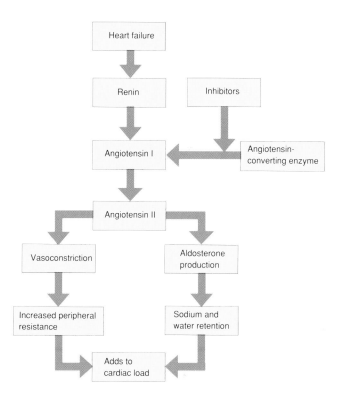

Figure 13
Effect of heart failure on renin release and the role of ACE inhibitors.

- Use a low dose of a short-acting agent as a test dose (eg, captopril 6.25 mg). Effect occurs in 90 minutes and will be over quickly. Hypotension responds to putting feet up and to fluid replacement.

- In clinical practice I titrate to effect at 3–4-day or weekly intervals (eg, captopril 12.5 mg bid, 25 mg bid and 50 mg bid), checking U & E at each increment.
  NB The data sheet, however, recommends titration with intervals of at least 2 weeks.

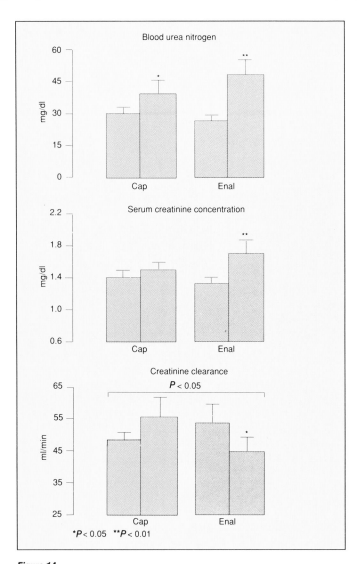

Figure 14
Comparison between the effects of captopril (Cap) and enalapril (Enal) on renal function – blood urea nitrogen, serum creatinine concentration and creatinine clearance – in a study of 42 patients with severe heart failure. The first column represents the control, the second the drug. (Reproduced with permission from N Engl J Med (1986) **315**: 852.)

- Longer-acting ACE inhibitors (eg, lisinopril and enalapril) may be used after the initial test dose of captopril out of hospital but should be initiated for safety reasons in hospital as first-time ACE therapy.

- Long-acting ACE inhibitors have a delayed-onset hypotensive effect which may be prolonged.

- Long-acting ACE inhibitors are more likely to have an adverse effect on renal blood flow (Figure 14).

- As output improves, diuretic needs may decline.

Other ACE inhibitor properties of potential value:

- Reduce incidence of ventricular arrhythmias

- Sulphydryl group may reduce free radicals and reperfusion injury and prevent nitrate tolerance

- May improve coronary flow at the same time as reducing oxygen demand

ACE inhibitors in severe cases:

- In hospital

- Low doses of short-acting agents initially

- SBP >90 mm Hg

- Closely monitor U & E

- If dry, reduce diuretics first

- Titrate cautiously (eg, 6.25 mg captopril bid for 2 weeks, then 12.5 mg bid for 2 weeks, and so on)

- Beware of hyperkalaemia if potassium-sparing agents co-prescribed

- If antihypertensive agents in use, reduce or stop as ACE inhibitors commence

- If moderate hypotension but no symptoms and good clinical response, continue ACE inhibitors

ACE inhibitors — adverse effects

- Hypotension: usually over-diuresed, dehydrated patients. Always use small dose of short-acting agent initially to avoid delayed effect. If hypotension occurs, raise feet and give iv fluids if necessary (unusual). Try reducing diuretic until patient gains weight and then try again.

- Renal damage: regular monitoring essential before and at each titration point, then monthly, then 3-monthly.

- Angioedema: 1 in 1000 patients. Some cross-reactivity. Therefore avoid all agents.

- Cough: 5 per cent of patients. Dry, non-productive and worse at night. Resolves 1 week after cessation. Class effect. Before attributing to ACE inhibitor check not due to pulmonary congestion.

- Toxicity to fetus: avoid in pregnancy.

- Skin rashes: 4 per cent.

- Disorders of taste (possibly more common with captopril), neutropenia, thrombocytopenia, aplastic anaemia occur rarely. ACE inhibitors potentiate lithium and chlorpromazine.

Nitrates

- Mainly reduce preload.

- Especially useful when failure due to underlying ischaemia and/or mitral regurgitation.

- Isosorbide mononitrate preferred to ISDN because of 100 per cent bioavailability.

- Dose 10–40 mg twice daily.

Table 7
ACE Inhibitors

Drug	Captopril	Enalapril	Lisinopril	Ramipril	Quinapril	Perindopril
Sulphydryl group	Yes	No	No	No	No	No
Prodrug	No	Yes	No	Yes	Yes	Yes
Half-life (hours)	1.8	11	12.5	12−27	2.5−4	12−24
First dose (test)	6.25 mg	N/R	N/R	N/R	2.5 mg	2 mg
Maintenance regime	6.25−50 mg twice or thrice daily	2.5−20 mg once daily or divided doses	2.5−20 mg once daily	1.25−10 mg once daily	2.5−20 mg twice daily	2−4 mg once daily

1 N/R = not recommended.
2 Prodrug needs metabolism to active agent which may lead to variable effects.
3 Sulphydryl group may be beneficial by reducing the effects of free radicals.

- Can be used with other agents (eg, ACE inhibitors).

- Side-effects include headaches, flushing and occasional tachycardia. Rarely syncope occurs.

- Tolerance (decreasing effect with time) more likely with frequent dosing regime, so use once or twice daily.

- No greater benefit from patch (5 or 10 mg) preparations than from oral agents, though some patients get night-time relief by applying patch before retiring and removing in the morning. Can be added in this way to oral regime.

Hydralazine

- Direct smooth muscle relaxant — afterload reducer.

- Combined with nitrates in high dose reduces mortality, but side-effects very limiting and regime rarely used.

- Bioavailability varies: 25−55 per cent.

- High doses needed — usually 200 mg daily — at which level

there is also risk of lupus syndrome. Check acetylator status at this level; if slow, reduce dose.

- Can cause angina, headache and postural hypotension.

- Reserved for when ACE inhibitor inappropriate or leads to adverse effects.

Flosequinan

Flosequinan is a mixed arterial and venous dilator which acts directly by attenuating inositol 1,4,5-triphosphate (IP_3) and protein kinase C, intracellular mediators of vascular smooth muscle contraction.

- Studies have shown acute and long-term increases in cardiac index and reduced filling pressure.

- When it is added to conventional therapy, exercise duration is increased and symptoms of failure decreased.

- Additional benefit is possible when symptoms continue despite ACE inhibitors.

- Headaches very occasionally limit usage; it is generally well tolerated.

- Tolerance is not observed.

- Dosage is 50 mg once daily.

- In severe heart failure a 100 mg dosage has been associated with increased mortality.

- A 50 mg dosage can be cautiously used if creatinine clearance < 20 ml/min.

Flosequinan is recommended if symptoms persist in spite of conventional therapy which includes high-dose ACE inhibition (eg, captopril 50 mg bid) and when ACE inhibitors are contra-indicated or lead to unacceptable adverse effects.

Calcium antagonists

- Calcium is essential for cardiac contraction.

- The more peripherally acting agents may offset any negative inotropic property by vasodilatation (afterload reduction).

- This approach carries risks not inherent with ACE inhibitors or nitrates, and with no proven mortality benefits they are therefore not recommended for routine use.

- Calcium antagonists, however, may be of value in diastolic heart failure, providing there is good systolic function.

- They may be of use when mild failure and angina coexist, but nitrates are safer.

- If a calcium antagonist is indicated, amlodipine, felodipine, nicardipine and nifedipine (having the least negative inotropic problems of the calcium antagonists) should be considered first. Diltiazem may be used with great caution but verapamil should be avoided.

- Felodipine is currently being evaluated in addition to enalapril: amlodipine is also being evaluated in heart failure.

Inotropic agents

Digoxin

Several trials have now established that digoxin is effective acutely and long term in sinus rhythm, particularly when there is cardiomegaly and a gallop rhythm. It may be used with all other agents and the average dose is 0.25 mg daily. Less will be needed with impaired renal function and in the elderly, and as toxicity relates in part to potassium levels these should be monitored at the commencement of therapy and regularly if other agents are being adjusted.

Digoxin does reduce symptoms, reduces hospital admissions and improves exercise ability, and when carefully used, side-effects are not as frequent as believed — in several trials hardly more than placebo. Digoxin has not so far been shown to lengthen life; trials are now in progress. Where heart failure and AF coexist, digoxin is essential therapy, as is warfarin. Digoxin carries no risk of hypotension or dehydration. Thus it has a place as an alternative to ACE inhibitors if hypotension is a problem, and has a place in combination. It should be used more frequently.

- In AF digoxin should be prescribed to control the ventricular response (see page 22)

- In sinus rhythm and mild failure it can be safely stopped after 3 months but in severe cases failure may relapse.

- Digoxin can be used when the patient is hypotensive.

- Digoxin can be safely added to diuretics and ACE inhibitors.

- Digoxin has been used in all mortality trials that confer a benefit but no evidence exists for digoxin alone. Trials are in progress.

Toxicity

Causes:

- Age-related reduction in renal function
- Hypokalaemia
- Anoxia
- Hypercalcaemia
- Hypomagnesaemia
- Drugs likely to raise digoxin levels: spironolactone, triamterene, quinidine, verapamil, amiodarone and nifedipine
- Hypothyroidism decreases clearance

Signs:

- Anorexia
- Nausea
- Brady- and tachyarrhythmias
- Yellow vision (rare)
- Facial pain (uncommon)
- Gynaecomastia (rare)

Blood levels (assay 6–12 hours post dose) normal 1.3–2.6 nmol/1. Always do simultaneous K^+:

K^+ normal:	digoxin toxicity >2.5 nmol/l (certain at 5 nmol/l)
K^+ < 3.5 nmol/l:	toxicity 1.3–2.6 nmol/l (ie, normal range) possible

Treatment:

- Stop digoxin

- Treat arrhythmias as needed

- Correct K^+, check Ca^+, Mg^+

- Digoxin-specific antibody 40 mg in very severe life-threatening situations

Xamoterol

This is a selective beta$_1$ partial agonist which was developed for mild heart failure in the hope that it would up-regulate beta-receptors whose presence diminishes as failure and intrinsic sympathetic stimulation increases. Given the pathophysiology of heart failure with inappropriate sympathetic and renin activation, it was a logical alternative or addition to the ACE inhibitors.

It has suffered from inappropriate patient selection and clinical usage and has fallen from favour.

It is effective:

- In mild heart failure (frusemide 40 mg) when ischaemia is associated, particularly anginal pain

- In diastolic heart failure

- In addition to digoxin

It should be avoided:

- In severe heart failure (mortality is increased)

- If bronchospasm is present

- If resting heart rate >90 beats/min

- If SBP < 100 mm Hg

The dose is 200 mg once daily for a week, then 200 mg twice daily. The patient should be seen at 2-week intervals for the first month to monitor effect. Hospital supervision is advised when therapy is being initiated.

Other inotropic agents

These are mainly available intravenously. Dopamine and/or dobutamine can be used occasionally in severe chronic heart failure, in bursts for 24–48 hours to allow time to gain or regain control with diuretics and vasodilators.

Dopamine and dobutamine have positive inotropic actions, with dopamine in low dosage ($<$ 5 μg/kg per minute) increasing renal sodium excretion. Both are sympathomimetic amines and may accelerate the heart, increasing oxygen demand which could be disadvantageous in the presence of CAD. They are also potentially arrhythmogenic. Use of these agents is outlined in the section on acute heart failure (see pages 20–24). Dopamine up to 5 μg/kg per minute can be used to avoid stimulation of peripheral alpha-receptors which lead to vasoconstriction and increased afterload, and this can be combined with dobutamine titrated to effect (range 2.5 – 40 μg/kg per minute). ECG monitoring is essential.

Oral agents exist which stimulate beta-adrenoceptors. However, long-term administration will be expected to result in diminishing effects because of down-regulation of the beta-receptors, and of course this aspect of therapy is not physiologically sound on the background of the pathophysiology of heart failure.

The phosphodiesterase inhibitors enoximone and milrinone are indicated for the short-term management of severe cardiac failure as intravenous agents, as is dopexamine, a selective catecholamine which avoids alpha-agonist activity and vasoconstriction and which may therefore be preferable to dopamine. They tend to be agents for a last-ditch stand in severe failure or a temporary post-operative problem. They are not currently first-line agents.

Milrinone:	indicated when conventional therapy ineffective. 50 μg/kg by slow iv injection over 10 minutes, followed by infusion at 375–750 ng/kg per minute for 48–72 hours.

Enoximone:	slow iv injection — up to 12.5 mg/minute. Initially 0.5–1 mg/kg, then 500 μg/kg every 30 minutes until response or total of 3 mg/kg given.

Side-effects:	include arrhythmias, hypotension, headache, insomnia, nausea and vomiting.

Dopexamine:	dopexamine is indicated for short-term administration in heart failure principally associated with cardiac surgery. It should be diluted with 5 per cent dextrose before use (may develop pink colour). Should be administered via a central line or large peripheral vein. Dosage: 0.5 μg/kg per minute. Increase to 1 μg/kg per minute, and then in increments up to 6 μg/kg per minute at 10–15 minute intervals.

Side-effects:	include tachycardia, tremor, nausea, vomiting and anginal pain. Dopexamine lowers plasma potassium and raises blood glucose levels, so appropriate action is advised.

The Prospective Randomized Milrinone Survival Evaluation trial (PROMISE)[*] comparing oral milrinone with placebo had to be terminated because of a 28 per cent excess all-cause mortality and 34 per cent increase in cardiovascular mortality in the treatment group. Oral phosphodiesterase inhibitors therefore have no role in the management of chronic heart failure.

[*] Packer M et al, Effect of oral milrinone on mortality in severe chronic heart failure, N Engl J Med (1991) 325:1468–75.

Beta-blockers

The use of beta-blockers is highly controversial. Theoretical advantages include anti-ischaemic effects, up-regulation of beta-receptors, reduction in oxygen consumption and anti-arrhythmic effects.

Whilst several studies in Scandinavia have shown improvement in NYHA class and exercise capacity, there remain no data demonstrating effects on long-term morbidity or mortality. It is possible that some patients will benefit from very cautious use of low-dose beta-blockers but there remains anxiety about the risks of hypotension and of exacerbating cardiac failure.

I suggest that, when angina and mild failure coexist, an echocardiogram is performed and if the ejection fraction is over 30 per cent, cautious beta-blockade can be tried. Nitrates represent a safer alternative or could be commenced before beta-blockade, perhaps to increase the safety of its introduction.

In pure heart failure without ischaemic pain the most compelling argument against beta-blockers is the compelling argument in favour of ACE inhibitors.

Anticoagulation

Many patients with heart failure suffer the consequences of pulmonary or systemic emboli due to intracavity clot embolization. Others may develop DVT and its consequences. Anticoagulation should be considered:

- When AF is present either intermittently or sustained: heparin in acute failure and warfarin when stable

- In sinus rhythm when output severely reduced and/or evidence of significant LV dysfunction (ejection fraction < 30 per cent) and atrial enlargement

- If echo evidence of thrombus

- If history of TIA

- Recent trials suggest same anticoagulant efficacy but fewer adverse effects with lower doses of maintenance warfarin therapy

Heparin:	20 000–40 000 units over 24 hours by infusion pump following a 10 000 unit loading dose. Monitor by activated partial thromboplastin time and keep at 2–3 × control.
Warfarin:	8–10 mg daily for 3 days, then maintain to keep INR at 1.5–2.0.

Anti-arrhythmic drugs

- About 40 per cent of patients with severe failure die suddenly, many of a cardiac arrhythmia.

- Ventricular ectopics are common in heart failure patients but no prospective randomized trials of treatment have shown benefit.

- Pro-arrhythmic effects are more common in severe heart failure, that is, drugs can exacerbate the problem.

- All anti-arrhythmic drugs are negatively inotropic to variable degrees.

- Amiodarone is currently being evaluated, as are automatic implantable defibrillators.

Amiodarone is the drug of choice for malignant ventricular arrhythmias and to assist in the control of atrial fibrillation because it is the least negatively inotropic. In a pilot study post infarction the 1-year survival in comparison to no therapy was improved when malignant ventricular arrhythmias were recorded and treated.

- Dosage is 200 mg tds for 1 week, 200 mg bid for 1 week, and then 200 mg daily.

- Monitor efficacy by 24-hour ambulatory ECG.

- Assess thyroid status.

- Be alert for the many side-effects which include photosensitivity, over- and under-active thyroid dysfunction, pulmonary fibrosis, ataxia and tremor.

- In view of the adverse effects do not use amiodarone without careful thought.

Diastolic heart failure

- Assess LV function on echocardiogram.

- If satisfactory systolic function consider
    1 Beta-blockade
    2 Calcium antagonists
    3 Nitrates.

- If LV diastolic pressure increased with dyspnoea, use diuretics and nitrates.

- If doubts about systolic function, use nitrates and diuretics first and consider adding beta-blockade or calcium channel blockers later. Xamoterol may be a cautious compromise.

- If hypertrophic cardiomyopathy and good systolic function use beta-blockade. Avoid arteriolar vasodilators if outflow tract obstruction. Also need to evaluate for ventricular tachycardia (24-hour ECGs), as amiodarone is of prognostic benefit.

- Diastolic failure may progress to systolic failure and the dominant clinical problem will need appropriate therapy.

Cardiogenic shock

General:

- Usually follows acute myocardial infarction with a virtually hopeless prognosis.

- Early coronary angioplasty may improve this but quick action is essential. Employ thrombolysis if coronary angioplasty is not available

- Exclude mechanical cause (echo essential): eg, VSD, ruptured mitral cusp.

Specific:

- Begin oxygen.

- Correct arrhythmias by DC shock rather than negatively inotropic anti-arrhythmic agents if possible. Amiodarone is the safest option but lignocaine and procainamide can be used cautiously and have the advantage of short half-life so adverse effects quickly resolve when therapy is stopped.

- Insert arterial line and Swan–Ganz. Swan–Ganz gives indirect LVEDP (Table 8).

- Insert urinary catheter.

- If no Swan–Ganz available rely on clinical findings and check radiograph (Table 9).

- If pulmonary oedema begin inotropes, and add vasodilator (nitrates) if SBP ›100 mm Hg. Target PA diastolic is 15–20 mm Hg.

- If no oedema
    1 Hypovolaemia — JVP low
    2 Right ventricular infarct — JVP raised.
  Give volume expansion to 500 ml. Swan–Ganz essential. Try to raise diastolic PA pressure to 15 mm Hg; then if SBP ‹ 100 mm Hg, begin inotropes (pages 52–6)

- Consider intra-aortic balloon pump only if
    1 Surgical option
    2 Reversible option (eg, drug overdose)
    3 Transplantation option.

- Protracted treatment only delays death. Establish your objectives clearly and if you fail to reach them retire gracefully for the patient's sake.

Table 8
Circulatory collapse: treatment based on simple haemodynamic assessment

Left ventricular end-diastolic pressure (mm Hg)	Blood pressure	Tissue perfusion	Treatment
>18	N	N	Vasodilator
	N	L	Vasodilator
	L	N	Vasodilator + inotrope
	L	L	Inotrope + vasodilator
< 18	N	N	Observe
	N	L	Vasodilator
	L	N	Possibly inotrope or no treatment
	L	L	Inotrope + ? Vasodilator
< 10	L	N or L	Volume expansion
	N	N or L	Volume expansion

N = normal.
L = low.

(Reproduced with permission from *Medicine International* (1989) **67:2794**.)

Table 9
Chest radiograph guide in cardiogenic shock

Appearance	Action
Normal lungs	Infuse 100–200 ml of normal saline or colloid over 15 minutes
Upper lobe veins distended or interstitial oedema	Begin inotropes and add vasodilator if SBP rises >100 mm Hg

Specific Areas

Surgery of heart failure
Transplantation
Rehabilitation
Terminal care
Practical points

Surgery of heart failure

It remains essential in the assessment of heart failure to exclude a treatable cause, in particular:

- Aortic valve disease

- Mitral valve disease

- LV aneurysm

- Post-infarction VSD

If any of these exists in the presence of severe failure, obtain an immediate surgical opinion to facilitate joint and therefore optimal management.

With ischaemic cardiomyopathy the role of surgery is more difficult to assess. It may have a more useful role when clear improvement in LV function occurs after ACE inhibitors demonstrating potential for surgical benefit (that is, reversibility). Surgery or angioplasty can relieve angina symptoms with a low risk if patients are selected carefully.

Thus an impaired left ventricle is *not* a contraindication to surgery but individual assessment is needed and precise, not vague, decision-making is essential. Though the operative risk may rise to 10−20 per cent when the left ventricle is impaired, long-term symptomatic and prognostic benefits have been established for bypass grafting when angina is associated with heart failure.

In hypertrophic cardiomyopathy, myotomy and mitral valve replacement may provide significant relief for selected patients with severe symptoms.

Cardiomyoplasty

Cardiomyoplasty is a newly developed operative procedure which involves wrapping the latissimus dorsi muscle around the heart. The muscle is dissected while its nerve and blood supply are kept intact. Two intramuscular leads are placed in the muscle and an epicardial or endocardial lead is placed on or in the ventricle. After 2 weeks the skeletal muscle is stimulated in synchrony with the heart to augment output. Early reports suggest low operative mortality and the potential for clinical improvement for up to 12 months.

Cardiomyoplasty represents an option for those with refractory heart failure who are ineligible for a transplant or as a bridge to transplantation when a donor becomes available. We do not know whether it will be an alternative to transplantation. The procedure is in its very early phases of evaluation.

Transplantation

Heart transplantation is still the only option for the unfortunate who have minimal LV function. It is a palliative procedure with many social and psychological as well as physical facets. The age level has increased from 50 years or less to good for their age people in their 60s. It is not a road to be embarked upon lightly, yet the benefits are potentially enormous and most individuals are prepared to put up with the rigours of monitoring and drug therapy for a chance to live and breathe normally again.

- Over 80 per cent are alive at 1 year (see Figure 15).

- 60 per cent are alive at 5 years.

- Improved quality of life is proven and without doubt.

- Rejection may be controlled with cyclosporin and monitored by cardiac biopsy.

- Accelerated coronary disease is the major long-term limitation and necessitates in the end a repeat procedure.

- Patients need strong social/psychological background to cope.

- Supply of donors limits procedure and ventricular-assist devices may be used to buy time. Similarly, total artificial hearts have been used as a bridge to transplantation.

Guidelines for selection:

- Age < 60 years (may vary if 'biologically young')

- Class IV symptoms

- Expected survival < 1 year

- Otherwise healthy

- Compliant, well motivated

- Strong family support

Relative contraindications:

- Associated systemic disease:
    'Cured' malignancies
    Sarcoidosis
    Amyloidosis
    Systemic lupus erythematosus
    Other collagen vascular diseases
    Crohn's Disease

- Active peptic ulcer

- Peripheral or cerebrovascular disease

- Insulin-requiring diabetes mellitus

- Psychiatric illnesses

Survival rates are as shown in Figure 15.

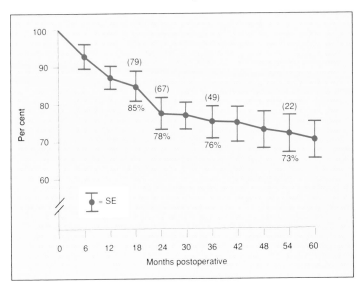

Figure 15
Heart transplantation survival (Johns Hopkins Hospital). The total number of patients operated on was 120: the numbers in parentheses above the points are the patients followed for that length of time; their percentage survival is indicated below the line.

Rehabilitation

Mild heart failure may, when controlled, only have common-sense restrictions:

- Avoid excess alcohol; do not smoke; avoid isometric exercise.

- Sensible dynamic exercise, walking, swimming, golf will be possible.

- Strenuous exercise must be avoided.

- Working (other than heavy labour), sexual relations, driving should all be normal.

Severe heart failure can be difficult:

- Activities must be restricted and the pace slowed.

- Stress must be avoided.

- Retirement on medical grounds from occupation is desirable if financially possible.

- Driving should only be undertaken if distress not easily involved.

- Sex can be safely enjoyed but the partner will need to be more active. ACE inhibitors used early may reduce the problems of impotence. Nitrates immediately beforehand may limit dyspnoea.

- Depression may need psychiatric assessment as a pre-existing problem may be present in addition to the more usual reactive depression.

- Advice and support may be necessary for spouses and children (of all ages).

Terminal care

Heart failure is a progressive disease and patients will at some point fail to respond to all our efforts. This can be distressing for both the patient and the family. It is difficult but important to know when to give up the struggle and to make the patient and the family as comfortable as possible. We have many techniques to buy time and they should all be explored, but there will come a time when an honest and positive decision to let the patient die peacefully will be the kindest option.

Practical points

With primary heart muscle failure we should consider ACE inhibitors early — certainly at the level of frusemide 40 mg a day and arguably at the level of thiazide therapy. These preparations are not difficult to use but must be avoided if the patient is over-diuresed. They can be safely initiated out of hospital following the guidelines I have outlined. With heart failure we now have a chance to make people feel better, as well as live longer. Our patients have options surgically and medically which it is a pleasure to realize — so it is essential that we make these available by being sure of the diagnosis and maximizing their treatment.

- Chronic heart failure implies that all correctable causes have been removed.

- Echocardiography is important in establishing that no occult surgical lesions exist and that muscle failure is the primary problem.

- ACE inhibitors improve quality and quantity of life in all classes of heart failure and should be initiated as soon as possible.

- ACE inhibitors may reduce the incidence of heart failure and benefit mortality when asymptomatic LV dysfunction is present.

- All vasodilators need preload and therefore the patients must not be over-diuresed before treatment starts.

- Diuretics must be monitored with U & E. Potassium-sparing agents are preferable when used alone but caution is advised when ACE inhibitors are co-prescribed.

- ACE inhibitors may be initiated out of hospital. Captopril should be used − without potassium-sparing diuretics at first. It is advised in mild−moderate cases only out of hospital (eg, ‹ 80 mg frusemide daily).

- Digoxin is essential with AF. Control may be helped with amiodarone.

- Digoxin in sinus rhythm is recommended when diuretics and vasodilators are not totally effective.

- In severe heart failure, anticoagulation may prevent embolization and venous thrombosis.

- No oral inotropic agents other than digoxin and xamoterol are currently available. Xamoterol is limited to mild failure only.

- Cardiac transplantation is an option for an increasing age range. Cardiomyoplasty may be an alternative.

- Hydralazine, combined with ISDN added to digoxin and diuretics, provides the only medical regime known to reduce mortality other than ACE inhibitors.

- Flosequinan may be of additional benefit if high-dose ACE inhibitors are not totally effective, and an alternative if ACE inhibitors are contraindicated or limited by adverse effects.

Index

ACE inhibitors *see* angiotensin-
    converting enzyme inhibitors
actin, 9
acute heart failure, 4, 12
    management, 20–4
AF *see* atrial fibrillation
afterload, 9
alcohol, 10, 15, 23, 25, 68
aldosterone, 8, 29, 44
allopurinol, 31
amiloride, 29, 30, 31
aminophylline, 21, 24
amiodarone, 23, 53, 59, 60, 71
amlodipine, 51
amyloidosis, 67
anaemia, 4, 11, 15, 23, 48
aneurysm, left ventricular, 17, 64
ANF *see* atrial natriuretic factor
angina, 13, 15, 50, 51, 54, 57, 64
angioedema, 48
angiography, 18
angioplasty, 61, 64
angiotensin, 6, 7, 8
angiotensin-converting enzyme (ACE)
        inhibitors, 26, 29, 31, 32, 44–8,
        57
    adverse effects, 47–8
    alternatives to, 51, 52, 54, 71
    beneficial effects, 44, 47
    guidelines, 44–5, 70-1
    and impotence, 68
    for moderate heart failure, 30
    in severe cases, 47
    surgery after, 64
    trials, 33–43
ankles, swollen, 13
anorexia, 53
anoxia, 53
anti-arrhythmic drugs, 11, 59
anticoagulation, 23, 24, 58, 71
antiemetics, 20, 24
aorta:
    aortic impedance, 9
    aortic regurgitation, 10
    coarctation of, 10
    intra-aortic balloon pump, 62
    stenosis, 10
    valve disease, 15, 64

aplastic anaemia, 48
arginine vasopressin (AVP), 6
arrhythmias, 11, 12, 17, 53, 54, 57, 61
    anti-arrhythmic drugs, 59
arteriovenous fistulae, 4
ascites, 14
ataxia, 59
atenolol, 24
atrial fibrillation (AF), 11, 12, 14–15,
        22, 23, 52, 58, 71
atrial myxoma, 11, 20
atrial natriuretic factor (ANF), 6
atrial septal defect, 10
AVP *see* arginine vasopressin

bacterial endocarditis, 11
bendrofluazide, 29, 30
beriberi, 4
beta-blockers, 11, 15, 23–4, 57, 60
beta-receptors, 54, 55, 57
blood count, 21
blood pressure, 15
bowel oedema, 14
bradyarrhythmia, 53
breathlessness, 12–13, 16, 26
bronchospasm, 21, 24, 54
bumetanide, 20, 28, 29, 30
    bypass grafting, 64

CAD *see* coronary artery disease
calcification, 17
calcium, 9, 27
calcium antagonists, 11, 15, 24, 51, 60
capillary pressure, 8
captopril, 45–8, 71
    trials, 39–43
carbenoxalone, 16
cardiac output, 6
cardiogenic shock, 4, 16, 61–2
cardiomegaly, 14, 17, 26, 52
cardiomyopathy, 10, 11, 64
cardiomyoplasty, 65, 71
catecholamines, 9, 27, 55
catheters:
    Swan–Ganz, 22, 42, 61
    urinary, 61
causes of heart failure, 10–11
chest radiograph, 17, 21, 61

chlorpromazine, 48
chronic heart failure, 4, 12
    management, 25–59
chronic obstructive airways
    disease (COAD), 20
circulatory collapse, 4
clinical presentation, 12–16
COAD see chronic obstructive airways
    disease
Co-operative North Scandinavian
    Enalapril Survival Study
    (CONSENSUS), 34–5
colchicine, 31
collagen vascular diseases, 67
compensated heart failure, 9
constipation, 25
constrictive pericarditis, 11
contractility, 9
coronary artery disease (CAD), 5, 10,
    12, 55
cough, ACE inhibitors and, 48
creatinine, 50
Crohn's disease, 67
cyanosis, 12
cyclizine, 20
cyclosporin, 66

decompensated heart failure, 9
deep venous thrombosis (DVT), 16,
    25, 58, 71
defibrillators, implantable, 59
definitions, 4–5
dehydration, 31
depression, 68
diabetes, 15, 16, 23, 31, 67
diamorphine, 20
diastolic heart failure, 5, 60
digitalization, 24
digoxin, 22, 23, 24, 26, 29, 31, 33,
    34, 52–4, 71
diltiazem, 24, 51
disopyramide, 11
diuretics, 26
    choice of, 29–30
    guidelines, 27, 70–1
    loop diuretics, 28, 29, 30
    management of acute heart failure,
        24
    management of chronic heart fail-
        ure, 25
    management of diastolic heart fail-
        ure, 60
    potassium-sparing agents, 29

side-effects, 31, 48
    thiazides, 28, 29, 70
    vasodilators and, 32
dobutamine, 22, 55
dopamine, 22, 55
dopexamine, 55, 56
Doppler studies, 17–18
doxorubicin, 11
driving, 68
drugs:
    causes of heart failure, 15, 16
    management of acute heart failure,
        20–4
    management of chronic heart fail-
        ure, 26–59
    management of diastolic heart fail-
        ure, 61
DVT see deep venous thrombosis

ECG, 17, 21, 22, 55
echocardiography, 15, 17–18, 21, 22,
    57, 60, 70
electrolytes, 21, 45, 47, 70
embolism, pulmonary, 16, 58, 71
enalapril, 46–7, 49, 51
    trials, 34–8
endocarditis, 11, 16, 18
enoximone, 55, 56
examination, 14–16
exercise, 68

facial pain, 53
fatigue, 13
felodipine, 51
fever, 4
flecainide, 11
flosequinan, 50–1, 71
fluid retention, 8, 12, 27
frusemide, 20, 22, 24, 27, 28, 29,
    30, 44, 54, 70, 71

gallop rhythm, 26, 52
glucose intolerance, 31
glyceryl trinitrate (GTN), 21
gout, 31
gynaecomastia, 29, 53

haemorrhage, 16
heparin, 23, 58
high output failure, 4
hormones, neurohormonal activation,
    8
HY-C Trial, 42

hydralazine, 32, 49, 71
  trials, 33, 35–6, 42, 43
hydrochlorothiazide, 29
hypercalcaemia, 53
hyperkalaemia, 29, 30, 31, 47
hypertension, 10, 15
hypertrophic cardiomyopathy, 11, 64
hyperuricaemia, 31
hyperventilation, 15
hypokalaemia, 28, 29, 31, 53
hypomagnesaemia, 53
hyponatraemia, 29, 31
hypotension, 45, 48, 50, 52, 57
hypothyroidism, 53
hypovolaemia, 61

impotence, 68
indomethacin, 31
infections, 11, 15
inotropic agents, 52–6, 61, 71
international normalized ratio (INR),
  23
intra-aortic balloon pump, 62
investigations, 17–18, 21
isometric exercise, 68
isosorbide dinitrate (ISDN), 21, 32,
  49, 71
  trials, 33–4, 42, 43
isosorbide mononitrate, 21, 32, 43

jugular venous pressure (JVP), 14,
  30, 44

Kerley lines, 17

latissimus dorsi muscle,
  cardiomyoplasty, 65
left heart failure, 5
lethargy, 13
lignocaine, 61
lisinopril, 47, 49
lithium, 11, 48
liver, distension, 14
loop diuretics, 28, 29, 30
lungs:
  basal crackles, 14, 15
  pleural effusion, 15
lupus syndrome, 50

magnesium, 27
management:
  acute heart failure, 20–4
  cardiogenic shock, 61–2

chronic heart failure, 25–59
  diastolic heart failure, 60
metolazone, 30
milrinone, 55, 56
mitral valve:
  mitral regurgitation, 10, 15
  mitral valve disease, 64
  replacement, 64
  stenosis, 11, 20
morphine, 20, 24
Munich Mild Heart Failure Trial, 41
murmurs, 15
myocardial infarct, 12, 16, 61
myocarditis, 10
myosin, 9
myotomy, 64

naloxone, 20
nausea, 53
nephritis, 4
neurohormonal activation, 8
neurohumoral changes, 6–7
neutropenia, 48
New York Heart Association (NYHA),
  12, 13
nicardipine, 51
nifedipine, 51, 53
nitrates, 21, 24, 48–9, 51, 57, 60,
  61, 68
nitroglycerin, 32
non-steroidal anti-inflammatory
  agents, 7, 11, 15
norepinephrine, 8

oedema, 13–14
  drug therapy, 30
  peripheral, 14
  pulmonary, 12, 17, 20, 61
opiates, 20
out-of-hospital care:
  acute heart failure, 24
  chronic heart failure, 25
  rehabilitation, 68
oxygen, 20, 24, 57, 61

Paget's disease, 4
papillary muscle dysfunction, 15
paroxysmal nocturnal dyspnoea
  (PND), 12
patch preparations, nitrates, 49
pathology, 18
pathophysiology, 6–9
peptic ulcers, 67

peripheral resistance, 9
phosphodiesterase inhibitors, 55
photosensitivity, 59
pleural effusion, 15
PND see paroxysmal nocturnal
    dyspnoea
pneumonia, 11
potassium, 22, 23, 52
potassium-sparing agents, 29, 30, 31,
    47, 70, 71
prazosin, trials, 33–4
precipitating causes, 11
pregnancy, 48
preload, 7–8
pressure overload, 10
procainamide, 61
prochlorperazine, 20
propranolol, 24
Prospective Randomized Milrinone
    Survival Evaluation trial
    (PROMISE), 56
prostaglandins, 6–7
prostate gland, 20
psychiatric illness, 67
pulmonary congestion, 5, 8
pulmonary embolus, 16, 58, 71 .
pulmonary fibrosis, 59
pulmonary oedema, 12, 17, 20, 61

quinapril, 49
quinidine, 53

radiography, 17, 21, 61
ramipril, 49
rehabilitation, 68
renal failure, 20
renal function, ACE inhibitors and,
    46–8
renin–angiotensin system, 6, 8, 9,
    43, 44–5
respiratory problems, 12–13, 15
restrictive cardiomyopathy, 11
right heart failure, 5, 61

salt, 15, 25
salt retention, 8, 12
sarcoidosis, 67
septicaemia, 16
sexual activity, 68
shock, cardiogenic, 16, 61–2
sinus rhythm, 52, 58, 71
sinus tachycardia, 6, 14

skin rashes, 48
smoking, 25, 68
sodium retention, 8, 12
spironolactone, 29, 30, 53
steroids, 11
stress, 68
Studies of Left Ventricular Dysfunction
    (SOLVD), 36–8
sulphydryl ACE inhibitors, 47, 49
surgery, 64–5
Survival and Ventricular Enlargement
    (SAVE) Trial, 39–40
Swan-Ganz catheter, 22, 61
sympathetic nervous system, 6, 9
systemic lupus erythematosus, 67
systolic heart failure, 5, 9

tachyarrhythmia, 53
tachycardia, 14
tamponade, 16
taste disorders, 48
terminal care, 69
terminology, 6–9
theophyllines, 21
thiazide diuretics, 28, 29, 70
thrombocytopenia, 48
thrombolysis, 61
thrombophlebitis, 23
thrombosis, deep venous (DVT), 16,
    25, 58, 71
thyroid dysfunction, 59
thyrotoxicosis, 4, 11, 15, 23
transplantation, 65, 66–7, 71
tremor, 59
trials, 33–43
triamterene, 29, 53

ulcers, peptic, 67
urea, 21, 27, 46, 70
urinary catheters, 61

valves:
    calcification, 17
    disease, 64
    replacement, 64
vasoconstriction, 6, 8, 12
vasodilators, 24, 26, 32–43, 70
venoconstriction, 8
venodilators, 27, 32
venous thrombosis (DVT), 16, 25,
    58, 71

ventricles:
    function, 7–8
    impaired filling, 11
    ventricular septal defect (VSD), 10,
        64
verapamil, 24, 51, 53
Veterans Administration Heart
        (V-HeFT I) Trial, 33–4
Veterans Administration Heart
        (V-HeFT II) Trial, 35–6
volume overload, 10
VSD *see under* ventricles

warfarin, 23, 52, 58
water retention, 8, 12, 27

xamoterol, 24, 54–5, 60, 71

yellow vision, 53